THE RICHARD AND HINDA ROSENTHAL LECTURES
2003

Keeping Patients Safe

Transforming the Work Environment of Nurses

INSTITUTE OF MEDICINE
OF THE NATIONAL ACADEMIES

THE NATIONAL ACADEMIES PRESS
Washington, D.C.
www.nap.edu

THE NATIONAL ACADEMIES PRESS • 500 Fifth Street, N.W. • Washington, DC 20001

NOTICE: The project that is the subject of this report was approved by the Governing Board of the National Research Council, whose members are drawn from the councils of the National Academy of Sciences, the National Academy of Engineering, and the Institute of Medicine. The members of the committee responsible for the report were chosen for their special competences and with regard for appropriate balance.

Support for this project was provided by the Richard and Hinda Rosenthal Foundation.

International Standard Book Number 0-309-9441-0 (Book)
International Standard Book Number 0-309-54643-5 (PDF)

Copies of this report are available from the National Academies Press, 500 Fifth Street, N.W., Lockbox 285, Washington, DC 20055; (800) 624-6242 or (202) 334-3313 (in the Washington metropolitan area); Internet, http://www.nap.edu.

Addtional copies of this report are available from the Office of Reports and Communication, Institute of Medicine, 500 Fifth St. N.W., Washington, DC 20001.

For more information about the Institute of Medicine, visit the IOM home page at: **www.iom.edu.**

The serpent has been a symbol of long life, healing, and knowledge among almost all cultures and religions since the beginning of recorded history. The serpent adopted as a logotype by the Institute of Medicine is a relief carving from ancient Greece, now held by the Staatliche Museen in Berlin.

"Knowing is not enough; we must apply.
Willing is not enough; we must do."
— Goethe

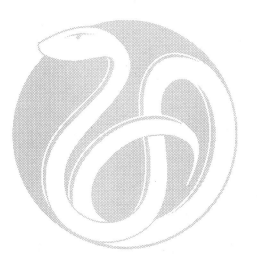

INSTITUTE OF MEDICINE
OF THE NATIONAL ACADEMIES

Adviser to the Nation to Improve Health

THE NATIONAL ACADEMIES
Advisers to the Nation on Science, Engineering, and Medicine

The **National Academy of Sciences** is a private, nonprofit, self-perpetuating society of distinguished scholars engaged in scientific and engineering research, dedicated to the furtherance of science and technology and to their use for the general welfare. Upon the authority of the charter granted to it by the Congress in 1863, the Academy has a mandate that requires it to advise the federal government on scientific and technical matters. Dr. Bruce M. Alberts is president of the National Academy of Sciences.

The **National Academy of Engineering** was established in 1964, under the charter of the National Academy of Sciences, as a parallel organization of outstanding engineers. It is autonomous in its administration and in the selection of its members, sharing with the National Academy of Sciences the responsibility for advising the federal government. The National Academy of Engineering also sponsors engineering programs aimed at meeting national needs, encourages education and research, and recognizes the superior achievements of engineers. Dr. Wm. A. Wulf is president of the National Academy of Engineering.

The **Institute of Medicine** was established in 1970 by the National Academy of Sciences to secure the services of eminent members of appropriate professions in the examination of policy matters pertaining to the health of the public. The Institute acts under the responsibility given to the National Academy of Sciences by its congressional charter to be an adviser to the federal government and, upon its own initiative, to identify issues of medical care, research, and education. Dr. Harvey V. Fineberg is president of the Institute of Medicine.

The **National Research Council** was organized by the National Academy of Sciences in 1916 to associate the broad community of science and technology with the Academy's purposes of furthering knowledge and advising the federal government. Functioning in accordance with general policies determined by the Academy, the Council has become the principal operating agency of both the National Academy of Sciences and the National Academy of Engineering in providing services to the government, the public, and the scientific and engineering communities. The Council is administered jointly by both Academies and the Institute of Medicine. Dr. Bruce M. Alberts and Dr. Wm. A. Wulf are chair and vice chair, respectively, of the National Research Council.

www.national-academies.org

Foreword

In 1988, an exciting and important new program was launched at the Institute of Medicine. Through the generosity of the Richard and Hinda Rosenthal Foundation, a lecture series was established to bring to greater attention some of the critical health policy issues facing our nation today. Each year a subject of particular relevance is addressed through three lectures presented by experts in the field. The lectures are published at a later date for national dissemination.

The Rosenthal lectures have attracted an enthusiastic following among health policy researchers and decision makers, both in Washington, D.C., and across the country. Our speakers are the leading experts on the subjects under discussion and our audience includes many of the major policy makers charged with making the U.S. health care system more effective and humane. The lectures and associated remarks have engendered lively and productive dialogue. The Rosenthal lecture included in this volume captures a panel discussion on the IOM report *Keeping Patients Safe: Transforming the Work Environment of Nurses*. There is much to learn from the informed and real-world perspectives provided by the contributors to this book.

I would like to give special thanks to Donald M. Steinwachs for moderating the November 2001 lecture. In addition, I would like to express my appreciation to Bronwyn Schrecker, Jennifer Bitticks, Jennifer Otten, Hallie Wilfert, Leah Small, and Shira Fischer for ably handling the many details associated with the lecture programs and the publication. No introduction to this volume would be complete, however, without a special expression of gratitude to the late Richard Rosenthal and to Hinda

Rosenthal for making this valuable and important education effort possible and whose keen interest in the themes under discussion further enriches this valuable IOM activity.

Harvey V. Fineberg, M.D., Ph.D.
President
Institute of Medicine

Contents

Introduction

ॐ

Harvey Fineberg

Good evening, everybody. Welcome. It is a pleasure for me to be able to greet all of you at tonight's Rosenthal Lecture.

For the last 15 years, through the generosity of the Rosenthal Foundation, we have been able to sponsor each year a talk or symposium which deals with a topic of immediate and lasting importance to health care. This year is no exception, and in fact it is a special occasion because today's lecture coincides with the release of our report, *Keeping Patients Safe: Transforming the Work Environment of Nurses*.

Now, it has sometimes been said that nurses are neglected. I have never understood that opinion because from my vantage point—occasionally as a patient, more frequently as a practicing clinician, and always as an educator—I have never failed to be impressed with the significance of nursing to health care, and that is not a sentiment that I am the only one to feel.

There is a wonderful expression of the importance of nursing by Lewis Thomas in his *Essay on the Youngest Science: Notes of a Medicine Watcher* in which he observes that hospitals are "held together, glued together, and able to function as an organism by the nurses and nobody else."

So, we are not here because there is a question about the fundamental importance of nursing and of nurses. Rather, the committee who dealt with the question about the work environment of nursing started with the question of how to enable nurses in hospitals and other health-care settings to function within environments that are safe and provide the highest quality of care for our patients. This is the motive for our analysis and this report, which follow a great tradition at the Institute of Medicine:

working on questions of patient safety and the quality of care. It is part of what we think of as our *Quality Chasm* series.

This is a study that looks simultaneously at the role of a very critical profession—nursing—and the function of key institutions, nursing homes, hospitals, other centers for health care. Because of this complexity, it was an effort that naturally called upon a wide multi-disciplinary group to look at and to try to understand the current work environment for nursing and what could be done to improve things.

I am especially pleased that the members of our panel agreed tonight to participate and to offer their reflections based on the report which has been released, but I want to take a moment before introducing the three who will be speaking to at least identify some of the others here who were members of the committee that produced the report. Andrew Kramer is professor of medicine and head of the Division of Health Care Policy and Research at the University of Colorado in Denver. Marilyn Chow is the Vice President for Patient Care Services at Kaiser Permanente. Pamela Mitchell is Associate Dean for Research at the University of Washington School of Nursing. Gwen Johnson is a staff nurse at Howard University Hospital in Washington, D.C. Mary Lou de Leon Siantz is associate Dean for Research at Georgetown University's School of Nursing. I want to thank all of you, and I am sure we all would like to join in thanking all of you, for your work in the preparation and completion of this important report. Thank you very much.

Now, it is my pleasure to introduce the first of our three speakers who will be sharing with us their perspectives on keeping patients safe by transforming the work environment of nursing.

The first speaker, who also chaired the committee, is Dr. Donald Steinwachs. Don is the Chair of the Department of Health Policy and Management at Johns Hopkins University's Bloomberg School of Public Health, and he is an individual whose own work exemplifies the kind of critical research in health services that is so sorely needed to improve the quality of care for all patients.

He has covered many topics, ranging from the effectiveness of care to the ways in which different organizational and financial arrangements may influence the quality, utilization, and cost of services.

As chairperson, his breadth of experience and scope of expertise were invaluable for integrating the many disciplines and vantage points that informed our report. It is a pleasure to acknowledge, to thank, and to introduce Donald Steinwachs.

Overview

෨

Donald M. Steinwachs, Ph.D.

It was a great pleasure to chair this committee and, as I will indicate in a moment, this was certainly a group effort that was very exciting. It was driven by a set of charges given to us by the funding agency, the Agency for Health Care Quality and Research, that asked this committee to identify the key aspects of the work environment of nurses that have an impact on patient safety and then to identify those areas where potential improvements could be made that would likely increase patient safety. As you know, an Institute of Medicine report is an evidence-based report, and so the recommendations you will be hearing, which came out of this work, are a synthesis of that evidence, an effort to try to pull it together in order to lay out a blueprint for health-care organizations in this country.

The committee's expertise—and you have met some of the committee members here—is unusual in the sense that it reaches outside of health care. We recognized there was a lot to be learned from organizations that have high reliability: those that have low rates of error. Industries that handle transportation, nuclear power, and chemicals have spent years trying to figure out how to avoid accidents. These are industries that are concerned with how to reduce rates of error by understanding human factors and engineering, the man–environment, and the man–machine interface. They recognize the limits of humans: that humans are fallible, that we all make mistakes, and that we need systems behind us to deal with these realities.

There is expertise here. On behalf of the committee, I especially need to acknowledge and thank Ann Page, who served as the study director.

She was the one who made this come alive and come together, and so some of us refer to her as Mother Ann, with proper respect.

And Janet Corrigan certainly gave a guiding hand to our work and helped shape the composition of the committee; at some difficult points she also helped guide the direction that we took.

Keeping Patients Safe builds on two prior reports. Harvey indicated *Crossing the Quality Chasm* and *To Err Is Human*, and very briefly to put it into context, *To Err Is Human* documented the fact that we have substantial errors that occur in health care. It focused on hospitals and in-patient settings, and errors that lead to the death of an estimated 44,000 to 98,000 patients a year. I think for most people it was rather shocking to think that so many people would die because of errors or accidents, despite the work of committed institutions and dedicated health professionals.

It addressed some regulatory policy issues that needed to be addressed. *Crossing the Quality Chasm* took a next step and focused very much on what the system needs to do to relate to the patient and to the actual delivery of health care, sort of the micro part of the system: what happens on the unit, what happens between the nurse, the physician, the patient, and other health professionals.

This report reaches out somewhat differently. It really focuses on the health-care organization and what hospitals and nursing homes need to do in order to address patient safety. It focuses on nurses, who are the majority of the health-care work force, who are the ones whom the patients see the most, and who are in the position to provide the kind of surveillance and monitoring as well as interventions, that are critical to patient safety.

Also, part of the *To Err Is Human* report was a clear message that humans always commit errors but that fundamentally if you want to reduce errors it is a system problem. You have to change the system. You have to build a system. In some cases, this requires redundancy to get reliability. In other cases it requires other structures to assure that when errors occur they are stopped immediately or they don't have a chance to occur at all. Most of the focus of this report is on the 90 percent of errors that are tied to failures in the system that are not really the blame of individuals.

As you know, nursing plays a preeminent role in health-care delivery. Fifty-four percent of health-care providers are nurses, and these nurses are frequently responsible for critical functions such as surveillance for rescue of patients and the coordination and integration of care. While all health-care providers contribute to errors, nurses often have the opportunity to intervene and to prevent that error from adversely affecting the patient.

The nursing work force, as many of you are well aware, is predominantly female. The average age of registered nurses (RNs) in this country is older than the average age of the entire work force, and so in relative terms it is a work force that is growing older.

Many of the nursing assistants, and we rely on them very heavily in nursing homes, are earning incomes that put them below the poverty level, and so this work force includes individuals who are working on the margins.

Some of the most disturbing statistics are those that relate to turnover. When 21 percent of hospital RNs leave their jobs during a year and have to be replaced, 56 percent of nursing home RNs leave their jobs and have to be replaced, and the same for 78 percent of nursing home nursing assistants, there are tremendous implications for patient safety and quality, which we will talk about.

We also recognize that part of nursing in this country is the use of temporary workers, and this report addresses their role and the related concerns that arise around patient safety.

When you talk about nursing today, many times the first issue is the shortage, and we will be talking about recommendations that deal with staffing and the relationship to safety and patient outcomes. In these recommendations, I think we have a positive message about addressing safety and improving patient safety. Many of the things that we will be proposing to you are those things that you would also propose to reduce nurse turnover and effectively reduce the nursing shortage.

Very briefly, there have been big changes in the eighties and nineties to health care and hospitals. We know that hospitals have gone through changes in payment, shorter length of stay, more acute patients. Nursing homes are seeing the same thing.

During the late eighties and nineties, there was redesign and restructuring, which affected the role of nursing in many hospitals and institutions and redefined that role in problematic ways.

At the same time, rapid increases in knowledge and technology have demanded that all health-care workers be able to master new technologies more often and use them effectively in order to prevent errors and problems for patients.

What you will hear about next in Ada Sue Hinshaw's presentation are the recommendations themselves and then the implications of those recommendations as seen by a CEO and hospital manager.

Management Practices, Work Force Capability, Work Processes, and Organizational Culture

ह▲

Ada Sue Hinshaw, Ph.D., R.N., F.A.A.N.

It is my pleasure this evening to be able to talk with you about the recommendations that came from the evidence and from the areas we had considered in terms of the blueprint for health-care organizations.

First of all, let me share with you the blueprint itself. Don was the mastermind of this blueprint, and we were all delighted with it because it brings it all together in one place, which is very helpful to everyone. Essentially, we are looking at threats that can arise to patient safety in four areas and strategies that we have looked at and recommendations that we have made in the same four areas: management practices, work force capability, work processes, and organizational culture.

Altogether, there are 18 recommendations, and 10 of them are primarily for the health-care organizations in the country.

Let us look at each of these individually but, first of all, let us take a look at management practices. Visible leadership, an interactive style, and decentralized decision making are all management practices that build strong and positive work environments.

We have seen this in a number of existing health-care management models in the country that have enacted this particular style of interactive leadership, which involves everyone in the organization—and particularly the staff nurses—in the decision making that is made with regard to patient care and staffing. Also, if leadership is not committed to the safety issues and to building the culture of safety, which we will talk more about later, then it is very difficult to improve safety in any way. In all cases, improvements should be made on the basis of evidence-based management, which develops strategies by relying on management research on how to form trust, manage change, involve workers, etc.

We have seen in the last several years some real differences and some real changes in hospital nursing leadership, and so it is important to summarize those. To say the least, they are familiar to many of the nursing leaders who are here.

The chief nursing officer has been given expanded responsibilities, but we don't know all the implications of this. There needs to be research to look at this particular issue. It could be seen as an opportunity for expanded control. It could also mean that there is less attention to be really given to nursing leadership within an organization.

As you look at the evidence of what has happened in the last several years, let me tell you that in one major survey in 1998, which focused on the chief nurse officers at university teaching hospitals, it was found that at 82 percent of the hospitals, the chief nursing officer has had expanded responsibility. In only 24 of those hospitals have we seen a shift in the nursing in their title, and only 24 percent now have nursing in their title. In some university teaching hospitals, there is no longer a separate department of nursing, and in 91 percent there was an obvious decrease in the number of midlevel managers who were available.

So, we not only have some major changes at the top leadership level; we have major changes at the midlevel management area as well.

The concern then is what happens with potential loss for a voice of nursing within those levels of management. Also, what happens in terms of the weakening of clerical leadership? Do we have in fact a number of people, a number of staff nurses particularly, who feel that there are no longer individuals available to them for intellectual and resource support?

Therefore, one of the first sets of recommendations is related to what health-care organizations need to consider in terms of acquiring nurse leaders for all management levels. From the top level of participation on the boards of health-care organizations to decentralized decision making with the staff nurses who are on the units, it is essential that nurses be able to provide consistent input and communication about patient care decisions and necessary health-care resources.

We also looked at five different management practices, and we particularly draw your attention to these because they are ones that are very helpful in terms of increasing safety for patients: first of all, balancing efficiency and reliability; secondly, creating and sustaining trust. This is trust in two directions. In other words, nursing leaders need to trust the competency, the decision-making capability of the individuals who are at the point of care. And individuals who are at the point of care need to know that their nursing leaders are in fact available to them, are concerned about their resource base, and have the ability to make their decisions move with patients, etc. Actively managing change is a very important part of this. We talked about involving workers and then creating a learning organization, an organization where the people share information; there is open communication; they are able to try new innovative ideas, study those, evaluate them and then have the feedback processes that allow the nurses and the workers in the organization to actually use that information.

With nurse work environments, there is evidence in the past decade and one-half of several areas that we are concerned about. Obviously, we are concerned about the increased emphasis that was on efficiency for a number of years rather than on the balance of efficiency with safety or with quality. There are also some issues of concern related to poor change management, limited nurse involvement, and limited use of knowledge management practices. As you can, there is an ample evidence base suggesting that these are some of the concerns in the work environment of nurses.

The next recommendation focuses on leadership at the top and the importance of educating all of the leaders, the board members, and the managers and about the idea of a culture of safety. We will talk more about that later, but the culture of safety is the link between management practices and safety, so that everyone is involved with the issues and the strategic planning around safety. For example, in a culture of safety, when a board member gets reports on financial affairs of the agency or the health-care organization, they also get a report on safety indicators and the outcome processes for safety.

The next recommendation deals with professional associations and philanthropic organizations, and looks for collaborations that will help health-care organizations to advance their evidence-based management practices. This involves putting together academicians and managers and nurses and the multi-disciplinary kind of team that was evident in our particular team, in order to think through together what we can do with management practices that will increase safety and make for strong and positive environments.

The next area in the blueprint is that of work force capability, and we looked at three different areas. Safe staffing levels are one area. As you know, there are a number of studies now that really help us to understand the relationship between nurse staffing and patient outcomes. It is very clear that when there is inadequate staffing there are negative patient outcomes, and we can talk in terms of an ongoing series of studies, from Kovner's earlier work in the late nineties through to Aiken's more recent work that was published in *JAMA*.

We also know more research must be done in the area of hospital studies. As we began to look at what we could do in the way of staffing recommendations, we ran into difficulty immediately because the studies, as well as they are done by Linda Aiken and others, are at the aggregated level of all units in a hospital or all nurses in a hospital. From this research, we could not sort out the separate medical-surgical component, and as Bill says, "What is a medical-surgical unit these days?" Research work really does need to be done to help us to better pinpoint what the staffing ratios need to look like or what staffing in general needs to look like in each area of the hospital.

We have better data in nursing home studies. For example, the data that came out of the U.S. Department of Health and Human Services (DHHS) minimum nurse staffing ratios in nursing homes was reported in 2001. Andy Kramer was a major part of that study, and so any questions we will refer to Andy. He has got this at his fingertips.

This is a very important study because it was very extensive, looked at a number of nursing homes and many patients, had very strong staffing data, and then found consistent associations between staffing levels and quality of care.

So, whether we are talking hospitals or we are talking nursing homes, the relationship between staffing and quality of care or staffing and errors in patient safety is very consistent and very strong. Essentially, this study suggests that there are persistent associations. He was even able to show that as you increase the staffing a certain amount you will get a certain increment increase in the outcome for residents, and if you increase the staffing again you will get a certain increment in the outcome for patients. So, it was very predictable in that sense.

There was of course a level at which the staffing was raised and there were no higher outcomes for patients, and so that provides very clear information about optimal levels of staffing.

It is important to note that more than 75 percent of nursing homes studied were below that optimal level. So, we have a long way to go in terms of the staffing issues with this particular area.

We took three different approaches in this area with work force capability, regulatory approaches that we are recommending, several internal staffing practices for the health-care organizations themselves, and a marketplace consumer-driven approach that we really liked.

It is going to be interesting to look at how we might move that particular set as well. First of all, we are recommending that the DHHS should update the 1990 regulations that specify minimum nursing home staffing standards. It was over a decade ago that these particular nursing home staffing standards were established, and at this point those standards called for a registered nurse (RN) in nursing homes only eight hours a day. We all know what has happened to the acuity of patients in the last decade and one-half. We all know that patients are going home or into nursing homes much more acute than they were, and the complexity of care has grown tremendously, and so it is really important now to look at and we are recommending that we require at least one RN within the facility at all times.

Currently, the standard for staffing levels and numbers is that there is one standard for staffing, and whether there are 60 residents or 300 residents in that facility that staffing standard doesn't change. That is the reason for the second staffing recommendation that we are making: the staffing levels really need to be changed as the number of patients is increased.

We then looked at staffing levels for nurse assistants who provide the majority of care in nursing home facilities. They are currently carrying about an average of 11 patients each, which is a very high number and does have some real consequences in terms of patient safety.

Let us now look both at hospitals and at nursing homes and some of the recommendations that we are making here. First of all, I don't know how many of you are familiar with hospitals in the sense of when they take their census, but usually it is at midnight. But during the day patients are admitted. Patients are discharged. Patients are transferred. All of this makes for extreme activity that the nurse must handle, and at each point, particularly transfers, the safety data show a higher risk for patients. We need to become much more aware of how many patients we are actually working with.

One study that looked at a medical-surgical unit found that during the midnight census they had an average of 23 patients, but when they looked at the full cadre of patients it was 35 on an average for that unit, 12 patients higher. You can believe that those patients were the ones being admitted, transferred, and discharged, patients who require high care.

With each of these you can see that we are moving to really look at getting direct care nursing staff much more involved in the decisions around staffing. Bill has a beautiful example he will use to show you that, and so I am not going to look at it much. We are also talking about getting elasticity into the system. It is going to be critical in the future for us to have some ability to have more staff or less staff as those numbers go up and down.

We also talked about direct care staff involvement and empowering nursing staff to regulate unit flow in that sense.

The other recommendation is for hospitals themselves and this is with respect to hospital intensive care units (ICUs). We were only able to make recommendations for the ICUs for the very reason that I cited earlier. In ICUs the research shows very clearly that once you have more than two patients the error rate does climb and complications occur. Take particular note of the way this particular recommendation is stated because what it says is not that this is minimal staffing or this is optimal staffing. Instead it says, "At any point the staffing gets to this level, you are at higher risk for patients having difficulty or having errors committed with them." So, if you have an ICU that has one nurse for every two patients, you need to become much more vigilant about what is happening with the error outcomes on that particular unit. It is the same for the nursing home recommendations that we have made.

We also looked at the recommendation for a nationwide system for collecting staffing data and have been particularly cognizant of the fact that it will take some time to get these data streamlined. There is some precedent with Centers for Medicare and Medicaid Services current in the Medicare/Medicaid service data.

There is nursing staffing data and so there is some beginning here, but we are also recommending that one of the things that needs to be built into the forthcoming hospital report card is staffing data because the relationship between nurse staffing and outcomes and safety is so strong. We are also suggesting that more time may be required and should be allowed in order to obtain this staffing data for the hospital report card.

Remember, we are also talking about knowledge capability and acquisition of knowledge, and this is something related to the educational and training recommendations that we are making.

It interested us that in most safety-sensitive industries there is quite a bit of money spent on training. When we look at health-care safety training in relationship to those other industries, we come up short and so it is important to note that data.

We then made a series of recommendations about assisting nursing staff in ongoing acquisition and the maintenance of knowledge and skills. These are not recommendations that you might expect, but they are very important to have made explicit in this report, and are even more important because of the need to enhance knowledge about existing and future technologies.

We next had several recommendations around the interdisciplinary collaboration, and we looked at collaboration broadly. We were asked the question about RNs and doctors this morning on the webcast and during the media event, and I have to tell you that we looked very hard at the different studies. We found that most of the studies showed that over 85 percent of the nurses were reporting that they had very strong positive relationships with their physician colleagues, and so at this point one thing we know is that relationship is very important. It is crucial, but there is no data at this point except for anecdotal data to support the negativity that often surrounds that particular discussion.

Next in the blueprint is the work processes section. You can tell that we looked at two different areas. This particular slide shows you the first of the data concerning fatigue, looking at scheduled and actual shift durations. We go from 1.5 hours through to 22.5 hours in terms of range. You can tell the schedule data in the lighter color and the actual shifts are very different so that that is part of the unpredictability in what is happening with nurses. The 1.5 person, the person working 1.5 hours came in to work labor and delivery. They did not have any patients in labor and delivery, and so this person was sent home. That all makes for a problem in the work environment and a sense of instability on the part of the professional nurse.

So, I think it is something that we have to keep in mind. You can also see that about 84 percent of the nurses worked between 8 and 12 hours consistently.

The 12-hour shifts with limited rest are called sustained operations. That is when you do 3 to 5 of those in a row. The error rates increase rapidly after 12 hours of work, and also as we know fatigue has some very nasty effects on our ability to problem-solve and do critical analysis and to react quickly.

So, we have recommended that states should prohibit nursing staff from providing patient care in excess of 12 hours per day or 60 hours during a 7-day period. This is probably going to be one of the more interesting recommendations in the report, but almost every safety-sensitive industry that we know of and that we investigated has put limits on the number of hours that the individuals involved in that industry can work, everything from transportation to nuclear power plants. The early work that is being done now with fatigue and nursing shows us exactly the same thing in that sense.

Some of the other work processes are inherently dangerous, and we know that because they are both high risk and they are high frequency, which is what makes a difference, and so you can tell very quickly the difference here.

I should tell you—and I think I am being defensive, so I will say that up front—but when you look at medication administration, nurses commit a large number of the medication errors. I should also tell you that we intercept 86 percent of medication errors before they ever get to a patient.

So, there is a good side and a bad side to this, but nurses are fallible like all other health-care professionals. Hand washing: you see the data on that. You can see the inefficient work processes, what happens with documentation, time spent hunting and gathering. We are all aware of that particular phenomenon and also the time that is used while involved in a number of non-nursing activities.

So, we have a recommendation then countering some of that particular evidence for health-care organizations, and to really help with resources to redesign or to design the nursing work environment with these kinds of work processes in mind.

We are also suggesting that we need a multi-disciplinary group that will look at problems with documentation, because these problems arise from several sources and we need to be able to get a better grasp on streamlining it and deleting some. That last was my own opinion. I will tell you clearly.

The last blueprint area is that of the organizational culture and the culture of safety. We are very committed to the essential elements that go into that culture. Every individual in the organization is going to have to be committed to that culture of safety. It must be a long-term commitment by the organization itself. Some of the literature and the research suggest it takes at least 5 years, if not longer, to get such a culture into place, while maintaining the legally required confidentiality of data.

These are some very specific recommendations that we have offered through the report that have to do with the culture of safety. The next is the National Council of State Boards of Nursing working with other colleagues to really begin to look at how they can discriminate between latent errors, as Don defined them earlier, and errors that are actually human or errors that involve willful negligence or intentional misconduct.

Congress needs to pass legislation so that in fact people can report errors and near misses in errors and feel confident that they will not be either sued or maligned for providing information that will improve patient care.

So, we are back to the major blueprint, and that gives you a series of 18 recommendations that we had worked through.

Evidenced-Based Management and a Culture of Safety

❧

William C. Rupp, M.D.

My job is to ask "Is this doable?" You have heard 18 recommendations. Ten of those belong directly to health-care organizations, and I would like to suggest that they are all doable, and I say that as somebody working in and helping lead a health-care organization.

No one recommendation is any more important than the others, but certainly there is going to be more press about such things as staffing levels, hours worked, and design of work. Yet issues about evidence-based management and culture are crucial if we are going to make a safer environment.

Management and culture are less tangible than number of hours worked, but they are a very important part of the safety. So, I want to talk about three very specific examples of how we can introduce and trust evidence-based management and how we can create a culture of safety.

I won't give the whole outline but just some examples of the kinds of things that can be done in health-care organizations. This comes directly off of recommendation 5.2 that we employ nurse staffing practices that identify needed staffing for each patient care unit per unit, empowering nursing unit staff—and I emphasize nursing unit staff—to regulate work flow and set criteria for unit closure to new admissions and transfers as nursing workload and staffing necessitate.

Now, Ada Sue referred to some leadership practices. It is our job as leaders to balance that tension between efficiency, safety, and making money for the organization so that we stay in business. If this were easy, they wouldn't need us.

Creating trust throughout the organization is a major challenge because that is how we get at that culture of safety, and I will give you a very specific example.

We have to actively manage the process of change, and there is a whole literature about managing change: such information as don't do an across-the-board change in your whole organization on day one. It is the role of pilots and gradual change in organization. It is involving workers in the decision making on issues around work design and work flow. As a leader, it means that I admit I don't have the faintest idea in most cases what happens at the sharp end of health care, at that individual point of care delivery, and going to those people and asking them the best way to do things and then finally establishing a learning organization.

Now, let me show you a specific example that comes out of my previous site. We called it a capping trust policy. Call it anything you want. It is the basic idea that the nurses on a unit determine on an hour-by-hour basis whether or not they can accept new patients either as new patients or transfers. Notice I didn't say the nursing supervisor; I didn't say the unit coordinator. I said the nurses on the unit, and it is done basically hourly, on an updating basis depending on what new patients have come in.

These hourly upgrades are made available to every unit just by using the Internet, and we basically rate each unit on a red, green, or yellow depending on how busy they are.

It is asking the nurses can you handle another patient, and if they say, "Yes," the unit is green, and if they say, "No," that unit is red, it means "We can't handle another patient." They don't get another patient no matter what. If there are five empty beds on that unit they don't get another patient. This means sometimes working with other hospitals to send patients elsewhere or transferring or working around, but it is respecting and treating as professionals the nurses who work on that unit.

Now, I have had hospital administrators say to me, obviously, "Well, you can't do that; they will cheat and stop working." My response is very simple, "If you really believe they would cheat, that means you would do that in that position." I simply don't believe it.

So, this is one specific example. We call this a capping trust policy. Now, it works into the whole culture of retention. This is the vacancy and registered nurse (RN) turnover rate at Luther Hospital in Eau Claire, Wisconsin, going back from about September 2002 through September 2003.

At the very end you will see the vacancy rate rise. That has to do with a decision to hire about 20 more RNs. So, it factors in, and there are some vacant positions, but notice that turnover rate. It is under 1 percent most of the time, and the vacancy rate is about 1 percent. That is because the nurses are happy working there.

Now, it isn't a single thing. It isn't just the capping trust policy. It is all the things we talk about in this report. There are market-based comparisons to make sure that we are in the market financially. We have a nurse recruiter. There is a recruitment pipeline management. We have an accelerated specialty orientation and education program. All of the things that are mentioned come together to make that culture, but my point is that it is a culture of trust, and it involves recognizing those nurses and listening to those nurses on the floor.

Actually, at Luther the only one who could overrule those nurses was me, and I never did that. I often had a physician in my office saying, "But I was up there and I saw an empty bed." The answer is, "Yes, would you like to be admitted if they just said that they can't do it safely?"

These are the reported medical errors on one unit back in about 1998 when we started collecting some of these data by month, and then we began a process of going out. The head nurse and I actually went around to every single unit on every single shift and said, "Do you know how important it is that we start finding out about these errors?" This had all come about after *To Err Is Human* came out and we looked around and said, "Gee, is that us? That can't be us." So, we went out and started asking the nurses.

We explained the fact that we won't punish you for these things, and in fact I will punish you if you don't tell us. What happened was we initiated this policy called Fair and Just, and the reported errors skyrocketed. Was that new? Of course not. They had been there all along, just nobody told us.

So, we started doing some things about that, various interventions. They came down some, but still remained quite high because people were telling us about more things that were happening.

We did a culture survey, which was very interesting, Fair and Just; we called it non-punitive initially. I like this term Fair and Just better, but we had a non-punitive policy. I can tell you that. I was the CEO.

One of my staff said, "Maybe we ought to ask the staff out there if we have a non-punitive policy." So, we surveyed nurses, physicians, pharmacists, and ward clerks; had several different scenarios that we took to them; and said, "In this scenario involving a near miss, a patient with minor harm, and a patient who died, what would happen to you?" Fascinating information. Only 5 percent said that they would even tell us about a near miss. It didn't happen. It wasn't an error. Why would I tell you? That means 95 percent of the time when things happened they didn't even tell us. Would they be criticized for an error? Thirty-four percent said, "Yes"; 23 percent said that it would be used on evaluations; and 76 percent said that there would be disciplinary action if the patient died. Remember I was the CEO of this hospital, and I could have told you we had a non-punitive policy. Staff didn't quite see it that way.

Going across, the ward clerks who were at the ultimate sharp end, 7 percent wouldn't tell us about a near miss. Seventy-seven percent thought they would be criticized for an error. Thirty-eight percent thought they were used on evaluations. Seventy-six percent said, "We are out of here if we make a mistake that harms somebody," and only 50 or 25 percent thought we had a non-punitive policy. It goes over all the way in physicians, of whom 85 percent said, "We will be punished if a patient dies."

Coming back to the old philosophy, as a nurse or as a physician I am trained that if I work hard enough and study hard enough I won't make a mistake. If a mistake happened, then obviously I didn't work hard enough or study hard enough.

So, this baseline survey got us going, and we continue to survey like this to see it improve as people understand that we really are after this reporting.

Now, just a bit of background about getting that culture of safety going, and then I close. When *To Err Is Human* came out, we went back to our organization and started looking at incident reports, interviews with a number of pharmacists saying, "Gee, we just heard about all this stuff that is happening; is it happening here?" We interviewed a couple of nurses and—who was doing this? It was myself and two other physician leaders; then we sat down and did some chart reviews.

On one unit, for 6 weeks we reviewed 20 charts a week in detail looking for adverse drug events now not just errors but adverse events. We found 5 per 100 admissions. We were flabbergasted; 23 potential adverse events per 100 admissions, 14 pharmacy interventions, and in those 6 weeks there were seven major adverse drug events. Not one got reported up through the system. Not one.

As we took apart that 6 weeks of data, what we found is that 56 percent of the adverse drug events happened at the interface. The interface was from home to admission, admission to transfer, as Ada Sue was talking about, and then discharge, 56 percent of those.

We put in place a very aggressive process to begin reconciling, so roughly 213 adverse events and potential adverse events. We started an admission reconciliation process guaranteeing that we knew what those patients were on once they got into the hospital. It required nurses calling home and getting somebody to go home and look in the medicine cabinet. It is complex, but we got to the point where we were 99 percent certain we knew what a patient was on when they came in the hospital. That dropped the adverse event and potential rate significantly.

We then put in one for discharge because we discovered that patients went home on our medications and continued the things they had been on at home, so that discharge reconciliation and then a transfer reconciliation took out a significant number of those errors. This is all very public information in the organization. Everybody understands this. They are very proud of this, and it makes it a much better place to work.

My message is that this is doable. There are a number of different ways it requires us as health-care leaders to think differently about our organizations and working with the multiple professional organizations, but those 10 recommendations are doable and there is data and management data to show that we can dramatically increase the safety of our organizations.

Discussion

&

DR. FINEBERG: You have heard a very compact summary, and I hope you will take the time to read the report. I think you will find it really outstanding in its depth and documentation, and it is readable. It really is, but our closing messages to you are ones that I think you will resonate to.

One is that we cannot afford to wait to act. You look back, and it has been four years since the *To Err Is Human* report. Progress has been made but not as much progress as needed. This is a clear blueprint for health-care organizations.

While we were talking in the past hour I did the back-of-the-envelope calculations, and if you take the rates at which individuals are dying because of errors that the *To Err Is Human* report said in the last hour 5 to 11 people died in this country because of errors. What this report tells you, and what Bill showed you in his own experience, is that those numbers could be substantially reduced through building systems and processes that take the potential for error out of patient care.

It is clear, too, that organizations, and Bill could have talked about this, are going to have to invest different amounts of resources to move ahead because each organization is going to have areas in which they have some strengths and some serious weaknesses, but I think there is a very positive message here that when you look at what you need to do to improve patient safety you are also addressing those issues that reduce nursing turnover. Turnover is expensive. The estimates in our report are anywhere from $10,000 to $45,000 per nurse. That is a huge amount of resources if you are talking about 21 percent of registered nurses (RNs) each year or you are talking about in nursing homes about half of the RNs each year.

These recommendations also produce greater patient satisfaction, along with a sense of well-being and a sense of feeling that the care system has actually cared for them and they have received better outcomes.

In our report we also tried to document using case studies of specific organizations, and some research supports the evidence that we had that there are actually some potential financial advantages. In general, when errors occur it costs resources, and if you look at the payment system for hospitals, overwhelmingly those resources that relate to complications and to more intensive interventions for individuals who have suffered adverse effects cost the hospital resources, and so society, the hospital, and the patient pay for these errors.

I think they chose me to do this, but the very final slide shows that you need an academic up here to know that an important purpose for every report is to lay out a research agenda. I think as you go through the report, even though it is impressive, the amount of evidence we have now, the gaps in that evidence are also of great concern. When we talked about staffing guidelines for acute inpatient hospitals, we only had the data sufficient to talk about a guideline related to intensive care units and not for all the other units. In nursing homes we are in a much better position because the research has been done.

So, let me just point to a couple of these and not take you through all of them. One is a very clear sense that we need to move ahead on research that measures patient acuity in ways that are useful in staffing and to use it in standardized ways across the organizations to be able to produce and share staffing data. This report suggests having staffing data available and hospital report cards and nursing report cards in ways that are useful as well to hospital managers, to nurses, and others who have to use that information.

Issues around fatigue—some of these don't go away. Shift workers who are working a graveyard shift and a swing shift pay a price for doing that, and we need to have ways to help workers and help organizations handle that in the best way possible. So, additional research that goes beyond what we have already is needed, and especially research into this concept of collaboratives: bringing together the hospital, nurses, academics, and others who are involved in evaluation to learn together how to build continually the information base about how to improve safety and then to take those next steps forward. In the best of worlds, we would have a fail-safe operation and be able to guarantee patients that we can do them no harm.

Let me close with that. I assume that we have time for questions and would welcome those and your comments about what this committee has done and where we need to move from here.

The floor is open, and we are eager to open up for wide discussion at this time.

PARTICIPANT: You pointed out yourself that 10 of the recommendations are for health-care organizations, and I think most of the folks in this audience, I would guess, are from the nursing community. So, my question is what are your plans to bring this report to the CEO communities and what would you recommend for all of us? How do we get the message? You are very enlightened, but how do we get the message to the unenlightened ones?

DR. FINEBERG: Not the term some of my staff have used. Why don't you start? Really I am happy you raised this question because, truthfully, if all that happens is a report that is talked about in a room like this, it is not going to have its purpose fulfilled. So, Don, why don't you start?

DR. STEINWACHS: I will be happy to start off, and then I was going to turn to Bill very quickly, who probably has the real answer, but it seems to me that the translation process to get this from a report into action is not only that we need to create a sense of public demand, if not public outrage, about the continuing problems we have in the health-care system, but we have to be able to provide the kind of technical assistance, the ways in which CEOs and boards will feel comfortable, for moving into what they see as a major change.

I think what Bill described to us is a huge transformation in an organization. Well, there are very few people who will take that on unless they feel they can be successful and it will lead them to the right end point. So, having an example like Bill and some of the other examples in this country are critical and being able to provide the kind of guidance through collaboratives and working together so it is a joint effort; it can't just be an instruction, but it has to be a joint effort.

Bill?

DR. RUPP: I don't have the answer, but I would hope that we first start some controversy with this report and get some discussion going. We actually probably haven't spent enough time saying what our plan is for getting this out to multiple sites, but there are a number of other areas that we can bring in as we begin to publicize this, the 80 different hospitals that are magnet hospitals, for example, that also have low turnover rates. Mine isn't the only one. There are a number of examples around the country that we ought to be publicizing significantly to get this kind of information out.

I come back to the research. For so many hospital CEOs, the data is still not there. We haven't done the research to show the dollars and cents outcome from this, and we absolutely have to get it over time.

DR. FINEBERG: Do you want to comment on this? It is such an important point.

DR. HINSHAW: Yes, particularly from the viewpoint of being a member of the Governing Council for the Institute of Medicine (IOM), because the IOM has been very concerned about dissemination and getting the information into the field and actually beginning to track what kind of impact we may have had with these different kinds of reports. Already I know some of us on the committee have been asked by Janet Corrigan and by Ann Page which groups do we need to get to first; how do we prioritize these groups; how do we get into their conference agendas; how do we get into their literature, etc., and really begin to get the information out. That is very consistent with the usual way that the IOM is really concerned about not just sitting on reports. It is really concerned with the translation piece.

MS. LUBIK: My name is Ruth Lubik, and I am a member of the IOM. I am a nurse midwife. I feel that there is a team member missing in the way that the report is presented, and that team member who should be very important is the public or the client. If you are going to reduce errors, it looks to me as though the client him- or herself plays as important a role as does the nurse or the doctor. Until we give and acknowledge the role that people's involvement in their own care decisions, until we acknowledge that they deserve that and have that it is very difficult.

I was in London just last week, and in the *London Times* there was a supplement about orthopedic errors and deaths and so forth, and page after page was published for the use of the public to look at and read. I know that the whole mention of the National Health Service in England turns a lot of people not only off but on fire. So, I mention that with hesitancy, but as a nurse midwife I learned very early that if I did not have the pregnant mother and her family sharing in their care that it just wouldn't happen. You wouldn't find the improvement we hoped that we would like to see. So, I guess my question is to Dr. Rupp and to the committee members and I do congratulate them on a very difficult task well done, is how involved were clients, consumers, the people who suffered, let us say, in the look at what is going on?

DR. FINEBERG: Thank you very much for the comment. Would anyone like to react to it?

DR. STEINWACHS: I think she took it to you, Bill, and I will be happy to reply.

DR. RUPP: The question is how involved were the consumers in the look and not as much as they should be. Our natural tendency isn't to always go there. The specific example I am thinking of is in my current organization. We put up signs in every hospital room saying, "We promise to wash our hands before touching you." The hospital, nursing, and medical staff went berserk. By the way, the data that we now have shows that hand washing has increased exponentially after doing that, but I think the point is that our natural tendency, no, we didn't have consumers on this panel. Should we? Probably, but didn't yet at this point. That is not a natural way that we go every time.

DR. FINEBERG: Any other comments?

DR. STEINWACHS: I was just going to add my support to the view that *Crossing the Quality Chasm* I think talks eloquently to the fact that it is not the system that provides care, and you are a passive recipient if you are going to have good care, and that it is the interaction just as you are talking about, and what we failed to do is to provide the tools and the information for consumers and families. This report does talk about report cards, though the research we have today sort of suggests that report cards sometimes influence the providers a lot more than they influence the consumer saying, "How can I use this to make a better choice? How do I know that that nursing home will be a place I really don't want to go?"

DR. FINEBERG: Thank you for raising a critical point.

PARTICIPANT: Yes, I'm with the National Center for Patient Safety. I practiced cardiovascular surgery for 20 years, and a couple of years ago I worked for Senator Kennedy as a Robert Woods Johnson fellow. The nursing shortage was one of my issues, and as I traveled around the country and spoke to a lot of nurses, I was concerned that at the time—if you think back a couple of years ago, Congress' focus on this issue was primarily about increasing recruitment, getting more students to go to nursing school, giving the scholarships and loan repayments, and so forth—I really thought talking to the nurses I knew from the work place and the nursing groups I spoke to around the country would uncover the real issue. And I congratulate you for focusing on the real issue, which is the conditions under which they work, and a couple of questions in that regard. Number one, why is that only 10 percent of the work force in nursing in this country is male? If you compare the private sector with the Department of Defense, 30 percent of military nurses are male. I asked them the question, and they said that it was about career track and opportunities to advance in their profession that are just not there in the private sector nearly as much. That was why a lot of males told me they were in the nursing profession. So, I think that is an intriguing question when you think about the work force, especially the alarming figure that 20 percent of nurses who are training and educated don't even do nursing right now.

The other question I wanted to ask, actually two other questions. What is it about magnet hospitals that have a much better retention rate? It has a lot to do with empowerment, at least that is what I heard, but what in specific terms could you speak to? My other question I forgot.

DR. FINEBERG: You might have a chance to think of it as you get the answer to the first two, but those are two very important points.

Ada Sue, do you want to take on the first question to start with, which is related to why don't we have men taking up nursing, and what is it about career paths, etc., at this point?

DR. HINSHAW: I think part of it is career paths and people not understanding the multitude of opportunities that are open out there for nurses. Many people still see only the stereotypical kind of response to nursing, and what they don't understand is you can be a nurse in many locations, many sites. You can go through many different kinds of educational programs. You can advance in administration, education, and in clinical specialty and staffing roles and stay at the bedside in those roles, but I think many people don't see that kind of array of opportunities. There is also the issue that it has been difficult to be able to get the salary and the pay of nurses to continue to increase over time. We have gotten the initial salary up more, but it is still true that you top out earlier than you do in other professions, and this affects both men's and women's selection.

The other issue is image. I think we have to talk about that being predominantly female at this point. It is very difficult to convince particularly young 18-year-old men that this is a profession that really provides a number of opportunities.

What we see is there are many more men entering the second career programs than in the initial generic program. These are individuals with a baccalaureate in another field who may have some experience in work life who then come back into nursing. Image is no longer the same issue as it is for the 18 year old, and so how we begin to deal with some of those kinds of factors is very difficult. I mean I don't have these answers for any of that except to know that I think we really do have to become much more explicit about beginning to look at strategies for that.

PARTICIPANT: Advancement means leaving the staff level nursing position and going on to advance practice nursing, or perhaps industry where the skills of a nurse are much needed and much valued.

DR. HINSHAW: Except some of the CEOs now are really beginning to look at clinical ladders at the bedside and not the old concept of a clinical ladder but new kinds of skills that will be required that will take new knowledge capability. You can advance, but you can advance in the expertise of caring for patients, groups of patients within a unit and staying close to the bedside, but that has always been a problem. I agree with you. That is a tough one for us.

DR. FINEBERG: Thanks, Ada Sue.
Bill, would you want to comment on what makes magnet hospitals magnetic?

DR. RUPP: No, I will let Ada Sue do that.

DR. HINSHAW: I seem to be the resident expert on these particular hospitals. These have been very exciting institutions that do both recruit easily, in fact usually have waiting lists and do retain nurses, and there are several characteristics that come through in the research literature, both Aiken and her colleagues' work and Marlene Kramer and Schmallenberg's work.
Those characteristics primarily have to do with adequate staffing, autonomy, and control of their own nursing practice, very visible leadership that has a trust for the staff workers and uses decentralized decision making, increased educational opportunities both formal and informal in the area, and a culture of very strong interprofessional relationships, particularly the physician-nurse relationship. This is very important for individuals, but this is also what you will find in the literature that makes these places magnetic and in fact they have better patient outcomes. That has been studied in Aiken's work.

DR. FINEBERG: Thank you very much.

PARTICIPANT: If you will allow me, I remembered my third question. It is very quick. I ask this of Bill Rupp. What, if any, strategies have you employed to either reduce or eliminate mandatory overtime, which is a real sticking point for the staff nurse, especially one who tries to have some other life and has kids to pick up after school and so forth?

DR. RUPP: The question is, how do you reduce mandatory overtime? We don't have mandatory overtime, though there clearly is a pressure to do that. It comes down to if we are doing that, if we are asking people to stay late, then units need to be red and we have got to stop taking admissions, and we can't keep piling onto that. There are times when you have a patient population. We have them now. We have to take care of them. That is the facts of life, but there is no sense then in adding onto that burden as we go along. We have the opportunity to hold up on electives and to move patients elsewhere.

DR. MARX: I am Eric Marx. I am the Associate Dean for Faculty at the Uniformed Services University which is the federal medical school, and we have a graduate school of nursing. I am struck by the importance of this work because of something which I think most of the people in the room are aware of, the recent imposition by the Accreditation Council for Graduate Education (ACGME) of the 80-hour work week for house staff. What I wish from a medical educator's standpoint is that this kind of basic research was done prior to the institution of that.

You are talking about 60 hours. We are dealing with 80 hours, the issue about transitions, the dependence now that we are looking to on nurses to cover it when we have really kind of shift work and I would suggest to you that, when you are talking about areas of distribution for this particular study, it is very clear for those of us who are trying to deal with this that without a true reorganization of the infrastructure of the facilities in which we deliver the care, simply playing with the hours is not going to be it. Because if you look to see how most teaching facilities have dealt with the 80-hour work week, all they have done is changed around the schedules. You know, they haven't looked at why a house officer really only spends 2.5 hours doing direct patient care and like the data you got spends 4.5 hours looking up things and another 2.5 hours where we are not really quite clear what it is. It is usually waiting for a staff person or moving a patient around or finding things.

So, I would suggest that the importance of this work clearly transcends the issue of nursing and really is the first clear-cut environmental study that I have seen that deals with the entire structure. So, I would tell you the one place that I would start distributing this to is I would make this mandatory through the Association of American Medical Colleges.

So, it would go to every single dean of every single medical school in the United States and be a topic of conversation for every board of regents because this clearly provides information that we desperately need in order to compensate for what is really a system in some trouble.

DR. FINEBERG: Thank you for that comment. In light of the hour and the number of people at the microphone I think we will have time to take a comment or question from each of those who are now standing, and then I think we will have to wrap up.

DR. SCHMIDT: I am Maddie Schmidt from the University of Rochester, and I would like to expand on the comments that Ruth Lubik made and advocate for the idea that there is another set of missing partners in this discussion and that is families, particularly for our most vulnerable hospitalized patients. I have become very sensitized to this by a recently completed study by one of our young colleagues where she has instituted an intervention for families of hospitalized elders where she has nurses working with families to contract to work with the nurses to prevent certain kinds of high-risk complications in hospitalized elders, for example, decubiti and acute delirium. The work that she has completed in a pilot study shows a direct impact of that kind of collaborative work between nurses and families in reducing those kinds of complications. She is now funded for an RO1 to continue that work, but I think we have got the potential there of folks who are sitting in the hospital environment who care very much about what is happening to patients, and more active engagement of them as partners in this patient safety initiative I think would generate a lot of positive things.

DR. FINEBERG: Thank you very much for the comment.

DR. GIBSON: I am Rosemary Gibson with the Robert Wood Johnson Foundation, and in some spare time wrote a book on medical errors from the experience of patients and families.

Two quick questions for you. One is in some of the more successful reports on making change. I think of *To Err Is Human*. There were numbers that rose above the din of all the dialogue we have in our public life and also the 3,000 kids a day that start smoking. Is there a succinct message that you have for this report that will similarly rise above the din that is catchy? Because I think that is the thing that really makes the work that you do so successful.

Secondly, have you ever considered with all the wonderful work you have done in *To Err Is Human* and *Crossing the Quality Chasm* (that you might) develop a lay version for the ordinary educated public and maybe put some of these together so that we can create awareness? There are certainly great CEOs like yourself, but what about all the others, the ones who are the laggards? I don't think you folks can fix it. I think it is pressure from the public, as the National Roundtable on Quality report noted. So, would you consider doing a lay version that could help stimulate that?

DR.FINEBERG: An excellent suggestion. That first succinctly stated but rather complex initial question, does anybody want to have a comment on that? Don?

DR. STEINWACHS: We have it down to a long paragraph. We have a ways to go.

DR. FINEBERG: Fair enough but an important point. The lay version I think is a well-taken point and is something we should do. We will follow up with you and with others on that because I agree with you. So much of what we do has to be interpreted and conveyed in a way that is relevant to the reader or audience, and this is a very well taken point.

DR.TOWERS: I am Jan Towers with the American Academy of Nurse Practitioners. I have two brief questions. I want to commend you on this. This is really wonderful, although you always do good work. So, I don't know why we would expect anything different. But one of the things in looking at this that I am wondering, did you look at or was there any thought to looking at the levels of nursing that are used in terms of preparation within these frameworks to see what kind of impact that has on patient care? Of course, I am particularly interested in advance practice nurses. Also is there any talk, and there probably is and I am just not aware of it, of expanding some of this kind of work to the primary care setting? I know we are meeting with physician groups in relation to trying to think this through, and it is very hard to get a handle on that.

DR. FINEBERG: Good questions. Comment or reaction?

DR. STEINWACHS: Let me take the second one. I have already forgotten the first question. I can only do one at a time, and I was thinking Ada Sue would need to answer the first one. In the primary care setting, it seems to me it is one of the areas where research needs to move. Sometimes, at least for the patient, there is a lot of ambiguity about is it a nurse, who is the nurse, and what kind of support occurs in those environments. Since doctor's offices have all sorts of staff but as you move into the outpatient arena, as the *Crossing the Quality Chasm* talks to, really the potential for errors rises tremendously and you are much more reliant on the patient and the family to be able to carry this out, and it is a different sort of system that needs to be there, but it is crucial.

DR. FINEBERG: Ada Sue, do you want to comment?

DR. HINSHAW: On the first one that you had raised, the different types of nurses and then the accompanying education that goes with that, we did not try to get into that question because it is quite frankly a huge issue in itself and so did not try to go there.

We really were looking with staff nurses and nursing homes and in hospitals particularly because that is where we had the data. What can we do with the work environments that will really help keep patients safe?

DR. TOWERS: So, are we dealing with a lack of data still in relation to that, or is it that this is another issue that probably needs to be looked at sometime?

DR. HINSHAW: It is a lack of data in terms of education, and it is also a lack of data in terms of different settings. In home care we had almost all data. It is an excellent testimony, but no actual data that we could work with, and that was also true in ambulatory care sites and in primary care, as Don suggests. So, we have some work to do.

DR. TOWERS: Okay, thank you. I would also comment that primary care is carried out by more than physicians and nurses. It is also nurse practitioners and other advanced practice groups, and I think there could be some real teamwork in working on some of those things.

DR. HINSHAW: As a dean who supports two nurse-sponsored clinics and three school clinics, I understand that concept.
Thank you.

DR. FINEBERG: Thank you very much.

MR. BAGIAN: I am Jim Bagian and I am the Director of the Virginia National Center for Patient Safety. One of the things I wanted to ask a question or comment on is the third from the bottom here about methods to help night shift workers compensate for fatigue, and I wonder if that is a bit too restrictive. The point is we heard comments before about using hours as a metric, and I think most of the industries that have really dealt with this find that it is a very ineffective and blunt tool.

In fact, many of us that were asked to comment on the ACGME working for eight hours said that it is foolish and shouldn't be done because you can make yourself feel good about bookkeeping hours. But in fact we feel that with the ACGME guidelines it is very easy to comply with the spirit of the rule and yet not—I mean with the letter of the law and not the spirit of the law—and the fact is when you go to why aviation really feels this is a failed strategy although they are always the ones that are looked at, there is quite a bit of research done on this and the move now for instance in aviation is looking at fatigue countermeasures. The fact is there are ways to monitor fatigue, and one size doesn't fit all. For example, certainly as you pointed out here very nicely, cognitive capabilities, visual, and things like that are the first to go. However, some things, such as can you start an IV or something like that, don't. You can also monitor by strategically managing a person that stays over or is forced into that and say, "You know what, you don't set up the IV pumps. You don't calculate drips, but you know what you can take vitals," instead of just saying that you can't do it because that is unreasonable and not really founded on fact. You can look at things like napping, strategic napping, using caffeine, and things like that. I think nobody has really done this in a coherent way thus far, and it probably is something that should be considered because it is really more effective at getting the end result you want rather than this blunt instrument because one of the reasons it has failed is 80 hours from when, from when you got up in the morning? You are coming on at night shift. So, you are up all day. You painted the house. You go shopping and now you show up at 12 o'clock. I don't think you just start the clock at twelve. There is 15 hours before that that you are not counting and yet you are in compliance with the rules and really haven't done much to help the patient.

So, I think the reinforcement of the third one to really talk about strategies and methods is probably more beneficial because the hour thing has been looked at for decades, and there are no good answers to that, I don't think.

DR. FINEBERG: An excellent point and thank you all for a whole series of wonderful comments, very thoughtful and very valuable to us.

I want to conclude by thanking our panelists and all the members of our committee and staff who helped make this possible.

DR. FINEBERG: Thank you all very much for being here.

Biosketches

ʲ▲

Ada Sue Hinshaw, Ph.D, R.N., F.A.A.N. (*Vice Chair*), is Professor and Dean of the School of Nursing at the University of Michigan. She was the first Director of the National Institute of Nursing Research at the National Institutes of Health. Her research interests include (1) professionals who function in bureaucracies, job satisfaction, job stress, anticipated turnover, and patient outcomes; (2) quality of patient caregiving; and (3) instrument development and testing, including measures of patient satisfaction, job satisfaction of nurses, and anticipated turnover of nursing staff. In addition, she has studied the use of ratio measurement techniques in building and testing the nurse and patient measures. Dr. Hinshaw is involved in a number of health policy activities. In addition to the Committee on the Work Environment for Nurses and Patient Safety, she has served on the Institute of Medicine's (IOM) Nursing Research Panel Parent Committee on Monitoring the Changing Needs for Biomedical and Behavioral Research Personnel. She has also served on a number of national review committees and policy commissions, including the Advisory Council for the Agency for Healthcare Research and Quality. She is past President of the American Academy of Nursing, and a member of the IOM and its Governing Council. Dr. Hinshaw coauthored the first *Handbook for Clinical Nursing Research* and a text on *Magnet Hospitals Revisited: Attraction and Retention of Professional Nurses*. She has received numerous honors, awards, and honorary degrees.

William C. Rupp, M.D., is President/CEO of Immanuel St. Joseph's— Mayo Health System and Vice Chair of Mayo Health System. Previously,

Dr. Rupp was President and CEO of Luther Midelfort in Eau Claire, Wisconsin. He led that institution's integration with Mayo Health System and Luther Midelfort's nationally recognized efforts and innovations in patient safety. He is a frequent speaker at Institute for Healthcare Improvement meetings regarding medical practice innovations. He is Vice Chair for Planning of Mayo Health System and has served in multiple community leadership roles in Eau Claire. Dr. Rupp is a practicing oncologist.

Donald M. Steinwachs, Ph.D. (*Chair*), is Professor and Chair of the Department of Health Policy and Management in The Johns Hopkins University Bloomberg School of Public Health. He is Director of The Johns Hopkins University Health Services Research and Development Center and Director of the Johns Hopkins and University of Maryland Center for Research on Services for Severe Mental Illness. Dr. Steinwach's current research includes studies of (1) medical effectiveness and patient outcomes for individuals with specific medical, surgical, and psychiatric conditions; (2) the impact of managed care and other organizational and financial arrangements on access to care, quality, utilization, and cost; and (3) the development of better methods for measuring the effectiveness of systems of care, including case mix (e.g., Ambulatory Care Groups), quality profiling, and indicators of outcome. He has a particular interest in the role of routine management information systems as a source of data for evaluating the effectiveness and cost of health care. Dr. Steinwachs is past President of the Association for Health Services Research (now AcademyHealth) and is Chair of the Board of Directors, Coalition for Health Services Research. He serves as a consultant to federal agencies and private foundations, and is on the Board of Directors of Mathematica, Inc. and the Foundation for Accountability.